INTRODUCTION

Tadalafil is used to deal with guys who've erectile dysfunction (additionally known as sexual impotence). Tadalafil belongs to a collection of drugs called phosphodiesterase 5 (PDE5) inhibitors. These drugs save you an enzyme referred to as phosphodiesterase type-five from operating too speedy. The penis is one of the regions in which this enzyme works. Erectile dysfunction is a circumstance wherein the penis does no longer harden and enlarge whilst a man is sexually excited, or while he cannot hold an erection. When a man is sexually inspired, his frame's regular reaction is to growth blood float to his penis to produce an erection. By controlling the enzyme, tadalafil allows to keep an erection after the penis is stroked by using growing blood flow to the penis. Without physical motion to the penis, inclusive of that going on at some stage in sexual sex, tadalafil will no longer work to cause an erection. Tadalafil is likewise used to treat guys who've symptoms and signs and symptoms of benign prostatic hyperplasia (BPH). BPH is caused by an enlarged prostate. Men with BPH commonly have issue urinating, a decreased float of urination, hesitation at the start of urination, and a want to get up at night time to urinate. Tadalafil will make these signs much less severe and reduce the hazard that prostate surgical operation can be wished. This medicinal drug is likewise used to deal with erectile disorder and symptoms and symptoms of BPH. Tadalafil is also used in both ladies and men to treat the symptoms of pulmonary arterial high blood pressure to enhance your capability to workout. This is high blood stress that occurs in the principal artery that contains blood from the right side of the coronary heart (the ventricle) to the lungs. When the smaller blood vessels within the lungs end up more immune to blood go with the flow, the right ventricle must paintings harder to pump enough blood via the lungs. Tadalafil works at the PDE5 enzyme inside the lungs to loosen up the blood vessels. This will growth the supply of blood to the lungs and reduces the workload of the heart.

Cialis is an emblem-name prescription medicinal drug. It's FDA-authorized to deal with the following in men:

Erectile disorder (ED), a circumstance in which you can't get or hold an erection

Signs and symptoms of benign prostatic hyperplasia (BPH), a

prostate condition that may reason issues with urination

ED and symptoms of BPH collectively

Cialis comes as a pill that you swallow. It's to be had in 4 strengths: 2.5 mg, 5 mg, 10 mg, 20 mg. Depending on your scenario and what circumstance Cialis is treating, you'll take the drug both earlier than sexual hobby or as soon as an afternoon.

Cialis incorporates the energetic drug element tadalafil and belongs to a set of medicinal drugs known as phosphodiesterase 5 (PDE5) inhibitors. For ED, Cialis relaxes the blood vessels main to the penis so that greater blood can circulate it. For

BPH signs, Cialis relaxes muscles to your bladder, permitting you to urinate extra without problems.

HOW TO USE CIALIS

Read the Patient Information Leaflet provided with the aid of your pharmacist before you begin taking tadalafil and whenever you get a top off. If you've got any questions, ask your doctor or pharmacist. Take this remedy by way of mouth, with or without meals, as directed via your health practitioner. Do no longer take tadalafil more regularly than once day by day. The producer directs to swallow this medicine complete. However, many similar drugs (instant-release tablets) can be split/beaten. Follow your doctor's instructions on a way to take this medicine.

The dosage is based to your scientific circumstance, response to treatment, and other medications you'll be taking. Be sure to tell your medical doctor and pharmacist approximately all the products you operate (together with prescription drugs, nonprescription capsules, and natural merchandise).

To deal with the symptoms of BPH, take this medication as directed via your medical doctor, normally once an afternoon. If you also are taking finasteride with this medication to treat signs of BPH, talk with your physician about how long you ought to maintain taking this medicinal drug.

To deal with erectile disorder-ED, there are 2 methods that tadalafil can be prescribed. Your doctor will determine that's the first-rate manner so that you can take tadalafil. Follow your medical doctor's directions precisely on account that your dosage relies upon on how you're taking it. The first manner is to take it as wanted, typically at the least half-hour before sexual interest. Tadalafil's impact on sexual ability can also last as long as 36 hours.

The second manner to deal with ED is to take tadalafil often, once an afternoon each day. If you take it this manner, you could attempt sexual hobby at any time among your doses.

If you're taking tadalafil to treat each ED and BPH, take it as directed through your medical doctor, normally as soon as an afternoon. You may additionally attempt sexual pastime at any time among your doses.

If you're taking tadalafil once day by day for BPH, or for ED, or for both, take it frequently to get the maximum benefit from it. To help you recollect, take it at the equal time every day.

Tell your health practitioner if your situation does now not enhance or if it worsens.

HOW HAVE TO I GET CIALIS?

Here are some suggestions for taking Cialis competently and efficaciously:

1) Follow safe, advocated doses.

If you'd want to take Cialis for ED, you've been given two options: You can take one of the higher-dose drugs on an as-wanted basis (simplest whilst you need to have sex), or you could take a smaller-dose tablet each day.

A 10 mg tablet is typically advocated for as-wanted use, though a few guys would possibly discover that a lower (five mg) or higher (20 mg) dose works better. According to studies, there may be no distinction in safety or efficacy among those two alternatives.

2) You can make Cialis work quicker.

If you are taking Cialis as needed, make certain to provide yourself plenty of time (because it takes up to one to two hours to kick in). Otherwise, you May's pace it up when you've taken it. If that's no longer running for you, you can do not forget taking a decrease-dose tablet each day. This might be higher if you opt to be more spontaneous. If so, make sure to take it on the equal time each day.

No count number which manner making a decision to take it, don't take greater than 1 dose according to day.

3) Watch out for interactions with different medicines.

ED medications combined with medications for high blood strain can purpose dangerously low blood pressure. Never take Cialis if you take nitroglycerin or every other nitrate medicine for angina or blood stress. These encompass:

Nitroglycerin sprays, capsules, or patches

Isosorbide mononitrate (Imdur, Ismo, Monoket)

Isosorbide dinitrate (Dilatrate-SR, Isordil, Sorbitrate)

Taking sure medications or supplements can reason your frame to take away Cialis from your device quicker, such as:

Phenytoin

Fosphenytoin

Carbamazepine

Rifampin

Supplements like St. John's Wort

If you're taking these medications, it's essential to continue taking them as prescribed; however taking them one after the other from Cialis can be useful.

4) Know the ability aspect results.

Aside from a prolonged erection, which is an emergency, feasible side outcomes of Cialis consist of:

Flushing

Headache

Nasal congestion

Heartburn

Back ache

Muscle ache

Additionally, sufferers taking Cialis every day may also revel in:

Sore throat

Respiratory infections

Cough

Diarrhea

UTIs

Acid reflux

Abdominal pain

You would possibly marvel how lengthy you can properly use Cialis. Right now, there isn't a maximum time frame for safely taking the medication. But because the years skip, you could start taking other medicines, which include blood pressure or antifungal medicines that could be dangerous if mixed with Cialis, Viagra, and similar ED tablets. Always be sure any healthcare issuer you see is aware of which you take Cialis so that your medications can be adjusted effectively.

WHO CAN AND CANNOT TAKE TADALAFIL

Tadalafil can simplest be taken with the aid of adults aged 18 and over.

Tadalafil isn't suitable for some people.

Do no longer take tadalafil in case you:

Have had an allergic reaction to tadalafil or some other medicines in the beyond

Are taking medicines known as nitrates for chest ache?

Have an extreme coronary heart and liver trouble

Have recently had a stroke or a coronary heart assault

Have low blood pressure or out of control excessive blood pressure

Have ever lost your vision because of decreased blood float to the eye

Check with your doctor earlier than taking tadalafil in case you:

Have sickle mobile anaemia (an abnormality of crimson blood cells), leukaemia (most cancers of blood cells) or a couple of myeloma (cancer of bone marrow)

Have Peyronie's disease (curved penis) or a similar hassle along with your penis

Have liver or kidneys problems

Have a heart problem – your medical doctor will advise you whether or not your coronary heart can take the extra strain of getting sex

WHAT SPECIAL DEFENSE SHOULD I OBSERVE?

Before taking tadalafil,

Inform your health practitioner and pharmacist if you are allergic to tadalafil, any other medications, or any of the ingredients in tadalafil drugs. Ask your pharmacist for a listing of the elements. Inform your health practitioner if you are taking or have recently taken riociguat (Adempas) or nitrates which includes isosorbide dinitrate (Isordil), isosorbide mononitrate (Monoket), and nitroglycerin (Minitran, Nitro-Dur, Nitromist, Nitrostat, others). Nitrates come as tablets, sublingual (underneath the tongue) tablets, sprays, patches, pastes, and ointments. Ask your health practitioner in case you are not positive whether any of your medications include nitrates. Your medical doctor will likely tell you now not to take tadalafil if you are taking nitrates.

Tell your health practitioner in case you are taking street drugs containing nitrates ('poppers') together with amyl nitrate, butyl nitrate, or nitrite while taking tadalafil. Your doctor will probably tell you not to take tadalafil if you are taking avenue pills containing nitrates.

You need to recognize that tadalafil is to be had beneath the emblem names Adcirca and Cialis. You need to simplest be treated with one of this merchandise at a time.

Inform your health practitioner and pharmacist what different prescription and nonprescription medications, nutrients, and dietary dietary supplements you take or plan to take. Be certain to mention any of the subsequent: alpha blockers which includes alfuzosin (Uroxatral), doxazosin (Cardura), dutasteride (Avodart, in Jalyn), prazosin (Minipress), silodosin (Rapaflo), tamsulosin (Flomax, in Jalyn), and terazosin; amiodarone (Cordarone,

Pacerone); positive antifungals along with fluconazole (Diflucan), griseofulvin (Grifulvin, Gris-PEG), itraconazole (Onmel, Sporanox), ketoconazole (Extina, Ketozole, Nizoral, Xolegel), and voriconazole (Vfend); aprepitant (Emend); bosentan (Tracleer); carbamazepine (Carbatrol, Epitol, Tegretol, Teril, others); clarithromycin (Biaxin, in Prevpac); diltiazem (Cardizem, Cartia,Tiazac, others); efavirenz (Sustiva, in Atripla); erythromycin (E.E.S., E-Mycin, Erythrocin); HIV protease inhibitors along with indinavir (Crixivan), nelfinavir (Viracept), and ritonavir (Norvir, in Kaletra), lovastatin (Altocor, in

Advicor); medicines for excessive blood strain; nefazodone; nevirapine (Viramune); different medicines or treatments for erectile dysfunction; different medications or remedies for PAH; phenobarbital; phenytoin (Dilantin, Phenytek); rifabutin (Mycobutin); rifampin (Rifadin, Rimactane, in Rifamate, in Rifater); sertraline (Zoloft); telithromycin (Ketek); and verapamil (Calan, Covera,Verelan, in Tarka). Your physician may also want to exchange the doses of your medicinal drugs or screen you cautiously for side consequences.

Inform your doctor what natural merchandise you are taking, especially St. John's wort.

Inform your medical doctor in case you smoke; when you have ever had an erection that lasted extra than 4 hours; and when you have recently had diarrhea, vomiting, no longer been drinking enough fluids, or sweating plenty which may additionally have precipitated dehydration (loss of a big amount of body fluids. Also inform your health practitioner if you have or have ever had pulmonary veno-occlusive ailment (PVOD; blockage of veins inside the lungs); any situation that affects the shape of the penis;

diabetes; excessive cholesterol; excessive or low blood stress; irregular heartbeat; a coronary heart attack or coronary heart failure; angina (chest pain); a stroke; ulcers in the belly; a bleeding sickness; blood circulation problems; blood mobile troubles such as sickle cellular anemia (a disorder of the purple blood cells), multiple myeloma (cancer of the plasma cells), or leukemia (cancer of the white blood cells); or coronary heart, kidney, or liver ailment. Also tell your doctor in case you or any of your family individuals have or have ever had an eye disease inclusive of retinitis pigmentosa (an inherited eye condition that reasons lack of imaginative and prescient) or if you have ever had unexpected extreme vision loss, specifically if you were informed that the vision loss became due to a blockage of blood waft to the nerves that assist you see.

If you are a girl and you are taking tadalafil to treat PAH, tell your medical doctor in case you are pregnant, plan to emerge as pregnant, or are breastfeeding. If you emerge as pregnant even as taking tadalafil, name your doctor.

If you are having surgical operation, such as dental surgical procedure, tell the physician or dentist that you are taking tadalafil.

Talk for your doctor approximately the secure use of alcoholic drinks during your treatment with tadalafil. If you drink a big amount of alcohol (more than five glasses of wine or 5 photographs of whiskey) while you're taking tadalafil you're much more likely to revel in sure side effects of tadalafil consisting of dizziness, headache, fast heartbeat, and low blood pressure.

If you are taking tadalafil to treat erectile dysfunction, inform your health practitioner if you have ever been recommended by means of a fitness care expert to avoid sexual activity for scientific reasons or if you have ever experienced chest ache all through sexual interest. Sexual activity may be a pressure on your coronary heart, especially if you have coronary heart disorder. If you experience chest pain, dizziness, or nausea throughout sexual interest, name your physician right away or get emergency scientific treatment, and keep away from sexual interest until your doctor tells you in any other case.

Tell all of your health care vendors that you are taking tadalafil. If you ever want emergency medical remedy for a coronary heart trouble, the fitness care providers who treat you will want to realize while you final took tadalafil.

THE END

Made in the USA
Coppell, TX
13 September 2022

82972115R00020